PEMF Th

A Beginner's 5-Step Quick Start Guide on How to Get Started with PEMF Therapy for Managing Stress, Improving Sleep, and Other Health Benefits

Disclaimer

By reading this disclaimer, you are accepting the terms of the disclaimer in full. If you disagree with this disclaimer, please do not read the guide.

All of the content within this guide is provided for informational and educational purposes only, and should not be accepted as independent medical or other professional advice. The author is not a doctor, physician, nurse, mental health provider, or registered nutritionist/dietician. Therefore, using and reading this guide does not establish any form of a physician-patient relationship.

Always consult with a physician or another qualified health provider with any issues or questions you might have regarding any sort of medical condition. Do not ever disregard any qualified professional medical advice or delay seeking that advice because of anything you have read in this guide. The information in this guide is not intended to be any sort of medical advice and should not be used in lieu of any medical advice by a licensed and qualified medical professional.

The information in this guide has been compiled from a variety of known sources. However, the author cannot attest to or guarantee the accuracy of each source and thus should not be held liable for any errors or omissions.

You acknowledge that the publisher of this guide will not be held liable for any loss or damage of any kind incurred as a result of this guide or the reliance on any information provided within this guide. You acknowledge and agree that you assume all risk and responsibility for any action you undertake in response to the information in this guide.

Using this guide does not guarantee any particular result (e.g., weight loss or a cure). By reading this guide, you acknowledge that there are no guarantees to any specific outcome or results you can expect.

All product names, diet plans, or names used in this guide are for identification purposes only and are the property of their respective owners. The use of these names does not imply endorsement. All other trademarks cited herein are the property of their respective owners.

Where applicable, this guide is not intended to be a substitute for the original work of this diet plan and is, at most, a supplement to the original work for this diet plan and never a direct substitute. This guide is a personal expression of the facts of that diet plan.

Where applicable, persons shown in the cover images are stock photography models and the publisher has obtained the rights to use the images through license agreements with third-party stock image companies.

Table of Contents

Introduction

Pulsed electromagnetic frequency treatment, often known as PEMF therapy, is an approach that uses very particular frequencies of electromagnetic radiation to enhance patients' overall health and well-being. On the other hand, the frequencies used in PEMF are supposed to be healthy, in contrast to the frequencies used in cell phones, which are thought to be detrimental.

A negative charge is present on the cell wall of every cell in our body. The cell wall is the outermost membrane. This charge normally hovers around -60 mV in nerve cells; however, the net negative charge of other cells can vary quite a bit. Nerve cells are the exception to this rule.

Potassium and magnesium are both essential components when it comes to keeping this negative charge inside the cells. Both of these elements contribute to the retention of these essential ions within the cell, which is why they are so important. Calcium and sodium, on the other hand, should be maintained outside of our cells since an excessive amount of either of these ions might disrupt the delicate equilibrium that exists between these ions.

This delicately balanced system may be properly managed with the help of PEMF treatments, which will contribute to an improvement in the patient's general health and sense of well-being.

In this beginner's guide, we'll take a closer look at the following subtopics of PEMF therapy:

• What is PEMF therapy?

- How does PEMF therapy work?

- Benefits of PEMF therapy

- Use cases of PEMF therapy

- Pros and Cons of PEMF therapy

- Side effects of PEMF therapy

- Risks of PEMF therapy

- Who should not use PEMF therapy?

- A 5-step plan for getting started with PEMF therapy

- Picking the perfect PEMF therapy device

So, read on to learn more about PEMF therapy and how to get started with this treatment.

What Is PEMF Therapy?

Pulsed electromagnetic field therapy, commonly referred to as low-field magnetic stimulation or LFMS, is a type of treatment that makes use of electromagnetic fields that are delivered from the outside to assist in the healing of injured tissue and the reduction of inflammation. This method of treatment has been utilized for the treatment of chronic illnesses including injuries and osteoporosis for a considerable amount of time.

The area of pulsed electromagnetic field treatment, often known as PEMF therapy, has expanded at a rapid rate over the past few years as researchers and medical professionals have become more aware of the numerous advantages that this technology can provide. The capacity of PEMF therapy to promote cellular health and enhance metabolic processes already present inside the body's cells is one of the primary reasons why this treatment is so successful.

It makes use of the fact that cells react to electrical stimulation by boosting the flow of oxygen and nutrients, which in turn speeds up the process of healing. The body can experience a variety of positive effects as a result of exposure to PEMF, including but not limited to enhanced circulation and the regeneration of damaged tissue. In addition, this kind of treatment is not intrusive, and it does not have any known adverse effects; thus, it is a good option for those who are searching for a method that is both safe and successful in treating a variety of medical ailments.

The Pulsed Electromagnetic Field (PEMF) treatment is a potent instrument for boosting cellular health and function because it works by capitalizing on the cells' electromagnetic capabilities. This treatment makes use of certain frequencies to bring about favorable changes in cellular metabolism and to lessen the effects of cellular damage.

These frequencies function by regulating disordered electrical impulses within cells, which are typically the consequence of stresses or environmental variables that have impeded the body's natural potential for healing. This may be accomplished by bringing the electrical impulses back into order. In addition, these frequencies can assist to strengthen muscle fibers that have become weak and increase nerve transmission, which ultimately leads to an improvement in the general health of the cell.

Cell membranes can have their maximum health and function restored with the use of PEMF treatment. This enables the cell membranes to re-establish order within the passageways that allow for the exchange of nutrients and toxins as well as the synthesis of proteins.

PEMF treatment is an extraordinarily potent instrument that, when taken as a whole, makes it possible to promote optimal cellular health and support healthy biological functioning at the most fundamental level.

There is still a lot that is unclear about PEMF, even though it is said to have several benefits. It is necessary to conduct more studies to have a deeper comprehension of this novel therapeutic approach and to evaluate its potential for assisting individuals in regaining their health and well-being. Pulsed Electromagnetic Field (PEMF) therapy is increasingly becoming popular owing to the amazing outcomes it provides while having just a minimal effect on the body.

How Does PEMF Therapy Work?

Maintaining cellular health is essential for staying healthy and active. Cells are the building blocks of the body, and keeping them in good condition is key to maintaining overall health. This involves a variety of different factors, including:

Vitamins: Vitamins are essential organic compounds that are critical for the proper functioning of our cells. There are 13 essential vitamins, including Vitamins A, B, C, D, and E. These vitamins can be found in a wide variety of healthy foods, including fruits, vegetables, meat, and dairy products.

One of the key roles of vitamins is to act as catalysts for various bodily functions. For example, Vitamin B helps to support the metabolism by aiding in the conversion of food into energy. Additionally, Vitamin A is important for vision as it helps to promote health

Minerals: Minerals are essential nutrients that play a key role in the health and vitality of cells. The body requires a wide range of minerals to produce energy, build tissues, and carry out various other functions. Some of the most important minerals for cellular health include iron, magnesium, phosphorus, and calcium. These minerals work together at a cellular level to keep energy pathways open, maintain healthy electrical signals within cells, and promote the normal functioning of organ systems.

Hormones: Hormones are chemical messengers that our cells produce to regulate various body processes. There are two main types of hormones: steroid hormones and protein hormones. Steroid hormones are produced in the adrenal glands, while protein hormones are produced in the pituitary gland.

pH Level: A healthy cell must maintain a specific pH level to function effectively. Our cells have an ideal pH of around 7.4, which is close to neutral and relatively alkaline. This optimal pH promotes the proper functioning of organelles, enzymes, and other important components of the cell. Any deviation from this ideal pH can disrupt normal cellular processes and lead to dysfunction and disease.

For example, if a cell becomes too acidic, it increases the risk of developing conditions like rheumatoid arthritis or cancer. On the other hand, if a cell becomes too alkaline, it may be unable to properly absorb nutrients or eliminate waste products. Thus, our cells must work hard to keep their pH in balance if we are to remain healthy and vital.

Severe surpluses of nutrients and toxins: When our cells are exposed to too many nutrients or toxins, their ability to function properly can be compromised. Excessive amounts of nutrients can cause overgrowth or create an unstable environment in the cell, which may lead to pathology.

Similarly, toxins in large quantities can overwhelm the cell and disrupt its critical functions such as regulation of metabolism, immune function, and repair processes. At the same time, these harmful agents can trigger autoimmunity and inflammation within the cell or elsewhere in the body.

Cytoskeletal components: The cytoskeleton is a vital part of every cell in our bodies. Made up of an intricate network of proteins, this complex structure acts as a kind of scaffolding that provides both internal support and external structure to our cells.

In addition, the cytoskeleton plays an important role in allowing our cells to change shape and move around, allowing us to move and respond to stimuli from our environment. Whether we are sitting at our desks or reaching for an object on a high shelf, the cytoskeleton helps our cells accomplish these tasks with ease and dexterity.

PEMF Therapy At Work

PEMF, or pulsed electromagnetic field therapy, is an emerging form of treatment that uses electromagnetic energy to promote cellular health. This unique therapy works by addressing several key factors that are known to influence cellular health, including vitamins, minerals, the pH level of cells, hormones, and the cytoskeletal components of cells.

One of the first things that PEMF therapy addresses are the vitamins and minerals present within cells. These nutrients provide the building blocks for all cell processes, including hormone synthesis and immune response. By interacting with the various vitamin and mineral receptors found on cell surfaces, PEMFs can ensure that each cell has access to essential nutrients and can function normally.

The pH balance of cells is also an important consideration in terms of cellular health. An abnormal pH level has been linked to several health problems ranging from cancer to autoimmune diseases. Fortunately, PEMF therapy works by improving the alkalinity or acidity level of cells through ion exchange mechanisms. By regulating these levels over time, PEMFs can help prevent inflammation and other chronic symptoms related to poor pH balance.

Another key factor in cellular health is the presence or absence of certain hormones like insulin or testosterone in cells. Many researchers have hypothesized that imbalances in hormones could be one reason why so many people are vulnerable to illnesses like diabetes or cancer today. Luckily, PEMF therapy can directly target these hormone receptors to restore proper levels within cells and regulate vital hormone synthesis pathways.

Finally, one last key factor that PEMF therapy focuses on is the cytoskeletal components of cells, which consist of proteins called actin and myosin that are involved in cell movement and contractility. When these proteins become damaged due to issues like oxidative stress or pollution exposure, it can impact cell function negatively and contribute to chronic conditions such as heart disease or arthritis.

However, by strengthening these actin/myosin complexes through electromagnetism, PEMF therapy can support healthy cell contractility without impacting overall metabolism or protein synthesis rates too much.

Overall, then, it's clear that PEMF therapy offers a powerful approach to promoting cellular health through electromagnetism.

Benefits of PEMF Therapy

There are many benefits to using PEMF therapy, including improved circulation, increased bone density, reduced stress levels, improved wound healing, better sleep, and anti-aging effects.

PEMF therapy is a non-invasive treatment that uses electromagnetic fields to stimulate the body's cells. It is effective in treating a variety of conditions, including chronic pain, arthritis, anxiety, and insomnia.

Improve blood circulation: One of the primary benefits of PEMF therapy is that it helps improve blood circulation. This is because PEMF therapy helps increase the production of red blood cells and improve the function of the circulatory system. As a result, this can help reduce the risk of conditions like heart disease and stroke.

Improve bone density: PEMF therapy can also help improve bone density. This is because PEMF therapy helps stimulate bone growth and prevent bone loss. As a result, PEMF therapy can help prevent or treat conditions like osteoporosis.

Reduce stress levels: PEMF therapy can also help reduce stress levels. This is because PEMF therapy helps increase the production of serotonin, which is known to help promote relaxation and reduce stress. As a result, PEMF therapy can be helpful for people who struggle with chronic stress or anxiety.

Improve wound healing: PEMF therapy can also help improve wound healing. This is because PEMF therapy helps increase the production of blood vessels and improve the function of the circulatory system. As a result, this can help wounds heal faster and reduce the risk of infection.

Promote better sleep: PEMF therapy can also help promote better sleep. This is because PEMF therapy helps increase the production of melatonin, which is known to help promote relaxation and sleepiness. As a result, PEMF therapy can be helpful for people who have trouble sleeping at night.

Anti-aging effects: PEMF therapy has anti-aging effects. This is because PEMF Therapy helps increase the production of collagen and elastin, which are essential for maintaining a healthy skin appearance. As a result, regular use of PEMF therapy may help slow down the visible signs of aging.

PEMF therapy is a versatile treatment that can offer many health benefits. However, it's important to note that PEMF therapy is not a cure-all and should be used in conjunction with other treatments.

Use Cases of PEMF Therapy

PEMF therapy has a wide range of potential applications, including the treatment of chronic pain, inflammation, and other chronic conditions. Read on to learn more about 12 use cases for PEMF therapy.

Arthritis: Arthritis is a common condition characterized by inflammation and pain in the joints. This can make even everyday tasks a struggle, limiting your mobility and affecting your quality of life. PEMF therapy is very effective thanks to its ability to target specific areas in the body where inflammation is present.

By regulating blood flow and stimulating cell regeneration, PEMF therapy helps to ease pain and stiffness while also reducing joint stiffness. It can also prevent further damage by improving joint mobility, helping patients maintain their range of motion over time.

Depression and anxiety: Depression and anxiety are two of the most common mental health conditions. While these disorders can have serious and debilitating effects on quality of life, they are also highly treatable. One promising treatment option is PEMF therapy, which uses electromagnetic energy to rebalance brain activity and reduce symptoms of depression and anxiety. Studies have shown that PEMF therapy can be extremely effective in decreasing both the severity of depressive and anxious symptoms, as well as improving daily functioning.

Fibromyalgia: Fibromyalgia is a debilitating chronic condition characterized by widespread pain and fatigue.

Due to its wide range of symptoms, it can be difficult to treat effectively. Luckily, PEMF therapy has emerged as an effective treatment option for managing the various symptoms of fibromyalgia.

Studies have shown that PEMF therapy works by reducing pain levels, improving energy levels, and soothing other common symptoms like headaches and difficulty sleeping. By targeting the root causes of fibromyalgia, PEMF therapy can help individuals manage their symptoms more effectively, leading to a better quality of life overall.

Migraines: Migraines are a form of headache that has the potential to be disabling. Symptoms of migraines include sensitivity to light and noise, as well as nausea. Traditional therapies can be useful in providing some relief; however, these treatments sometimes come with undesirable side effects, which makes them less than ideal.

PEMF therapy is particularly successful at limiting the frequency of migraine headaches as well as the severity of those headaches. This is achieved by reducing inflammation and increasing blood flow to the brain.

Osteoporosis: Osteoporosis is a serious health condition that affects millions of people worldwide. Characterized by decreased bone density and an increased risk of fractures, osteoporosis places a significant burden on those who suffer from it.

PEMF therapy involves exposure to low-frequency electromagnetic fields, which have been shown to increase bone density and reduce the risk of fractures. Thus, PEMF therapy represents an invaluable tool in the fight against this debilitating disease, offering hope to those who are living with its harmful effects on their bodies and quality of life.

Sleep disorders: Sleep problems are a widespread and significant condition that can have a negative influence on a person's general quality of life, as well as their physical and emotional well-being. People who have trouble sleeping regularly frequently battle with symptoms that include feelings of weariness, decreased focus, and even mood changes. In addition, regular interruptions in sleep patterns have been linked to the development of long-term medical disorders such as anxiety, depression, and obesity.

In PEMF therapy, the body is subjected to an electromagnetic field with pulsing frequencies meant to promote different internal activities. One of these functions is the generation of melatonin, which is a hormone that is important for regulating sleep. PEMF therapy provides a solution that is both safe and effective for a wide variety of common sleep problems. This therapy works by enhancing both the quality and quantity of sleep.

Parkinson's disease: Parkinson's disease is an illness that is chronic and progresses over time. It is characterized by movement problems caused by a disruption in the brain's capacity to govern motor processes. This can lead to symptoms such as tremors, trouble walking, problems with balance, difficulty speaking, and stiffness in the muscles.

The use of pulsed electromagnetic fields, or PEMF treatment, to treat particular parts of the body to enhance blood flow and cell function includes the use of electromagnetic fields. PEMF therapy has been demonstrated to effectively reduce tremors, enhance mobility and coordination, and improve the quality of life for persons living with Parkinson's disease through this method. PEMF therapy also improves the overall health of patients.

Alzheimer's disease: Alzheimer's disease is an insidious condition that slowly erodes one's cognitive function over time. This chronic disorder manifests in memory loss, difficulty with problem-solving, and changes in behavior that can be devastating for patients and their loved ones.

Fortunately, there is a relief to be had in the form of PEMF therapy. This innovative treatment uses pulsed electromagnetic fields to enhance neuronal activity, improving cognitive function and helping to mitigate some of the symptoms associated with Alzheimer's disease. Extensive research has shown that PEMF therapy has the potential to reduce the likelihood of cognitive decline or dementia in those at high risk for these conditions.

Cardiovascular diseases: Cardiovascular diseases are conditions that affect the heart and the blood vessels that carry blood throughout the body. By slowing or stopping the circulation of blood throughout the body, these conditions, which include hypertension, high cholesterol, and atherosclerosis, contribute to an increased likelihood of suffering a heart attack or a stroke.

The Pulsed Electromagnetic Field (PEMF) therapy uses electromagnetic pulses to improve blood circulation, strengthen blood vessels and muscle tissue, reduce inflammation in arteries and other tissues, and stimulate the formation of healthy tissue. Improving circulation throughout the body, boosting heart health, and reducing the damage caused by oxidative stress, reduces the risk of having a heart attack or a stroke in the long run.

Cancer: Cancer refers to a set of diseases that are characterized by one another by the out-of-control proliferation and division of cells. Cancer is a complicated category of disease. Even while tremendous headway has been achieved in recent years by medical research in understanding the disease, there has been very little advancement made in the treatment of cancer. On the other hand, the process known as PEMF therapy has the potential to be used in the treatment of cancer.

In PEMF therapy, certain electromagnetic frequencies are used to hone in on cancer cells and induce the death of those cells by apoptosis. This occurs without impacting the body's healthy cells, which are not affected by the therapy.

In addition, research shows that treatment with PEMF can reduce the size of tumors by decreasing the quantity of blood flow that is required for the creation of malignant growths. This is accomplished by targeting the magnetic fields that are emitted by the device. Patients with cancer who undergo treatment with pulsed electromagnetic fields (PEMF) may see a considerable improvement in their quality of life following the treatment.

Despite this, you should seek the advice of an experienced medical professional to determine which approach to therapy will be most successful for your condition.

Chronic fatigue syndrome: People who have chronic fatigue syndrome, often known as CFS, may find that the condition makes it impossible for them to function normally. CFS is typically characterized by an extreme and persistent weariness that does not improve with rest or sleep, which can have a substantial impact on the quality of life of a person who is afflicted with the condition.

Nevertheless, there is a glimmer of hope for those who suffer from this ailment: a recent study reveals that PEMF therapy may be an effective therapeutic option for this condition. PEMF therapy makes use of electromagnetic fields to stimulate the activity of cells and tissues, which, in turn, improves the performance of the circulatory system, lessens feelings of fatigue, and generally raises the bar for overall quality of life.

Bladder and pelvic pain: Bladder and pelvic pain are two prevalent disorders that can be incapacitating and impede daily activities. These disorders may have a variety of underlying causes, such as bladder and surrounding organ issues or nerve injury.

PEMF treatment has been shown to considerably lower pain levels and enhances the quality of life in patients with bladder or pelvic discomfort by encouraging cell regeneration and decreasing inflammation in the afflicted area. Regular PEMF therapy sessions, whether used alone or in conjunction with other therapies, can help individuals regain the capacity to live without chronic discomfort or interruption from their symptoms.

Menstrual cramps: Menstrual cramps are a type of discomfort that can occur during menstruation and are often present in the lower abdomen. As this type of pain may be rather acute and might interfere with daily activities, it compels many women to seek therapy in the hopes of obtaining relief.

Menstrual cramps are effectively treated by PEMF therapy. PEMF treatment is the application of magnetic fields to particular locations of the body to relieve pain and create relaxation. These tailored fields lessen painful muscle spasms and increase blood flow, two frequent variables that contribute to the misery of menstrual cramps.

Pulsed electromagnetic frequency therapy is a non-invasive, drug-free method of treatment. It utilizes magnetic fields to speed up cellular repair and enhance healing. This method of treatment has numerous potential applications, including the treatment of chronic pain, inflammation, anxiety, depression, fibromyalgia, migraines, osteoporosis, sleep disorders, Parkinson's disease, Alzheimer's disease, cardiovascular diseases, cancer, chronic fatigue syndrome, bladder/pelvic pain, and menstrual cramps. If you suspect that this therapy might be useful for you, you should discuss it with your primary care physician or another certified medical practitioner.

Pros and Cons of PEMF Therapy

While there are many pros to PEMF therapy and it can be an effective alternative treatment in some cases, it is important to carefully weigh the risks and benefits before choosing this option.

Pros

PEMF therapy is a low-risk, non-invasive treatment that can be used as a complementary or alternative treatment for a variety of conditions.

Low-Risk Treatment: PEMF therapy, also known as pulsed electromagnetic field therapy, is a form of treatment that makes use of electromagnetic fields to repair the body and alleviate the symptoms of sickness and illness.

PEMF therapy, in contrast to many other medical therapies, carries a remarkably low risk and is associated with an extremely limited number of adverse effects and problems. This is due, in part, to the fact that the PEMF therapy does not include any procedures or drugs that might potentially lead to unintended responses in the body.

Can Be Used as a Complementary or Alternative Treatment: PEMF, or pulsed electromagnetic field therapy, is a versatile kind of treatment that has been found to offer a wide range of advantages for both physical and mental health.

As a complementary treatment, PEMF is commonly applied to other medical procedures to promote the healing process. For instance, it can be used in conjunction with conventional pharmaceutical drugs to lessen nausea that comes with chemotherapy treatments, or it might be used to boost the efficacy of surgery and physical therapy in the process of recuperating from an injury.

Alternatively, as an alternate therapy, PEMF can also be utilized on its own in cases when normal medical procedures might not be possible. Patients who suffer from chronic pain problems such as fibromyalgia, for instance, may discover that PEMF therapy provides relief without the hazards associated with drugs such as opioids.

Non-Invasive Treatment: Pulsed electromagnetic field therapy, often known as PEMF therapy, is a non-invasive kind of medical treatment that can help alleviate pain and speed up the healing process. PEMF, in contrast to more conventional therapies such as medicine for pain or surgery, does not place the patient in any danger or expose them to any harm.

Instead, it makes use of certain electromagnetic fields to activate cells, which in turn encourages the production of feel-good neurotransmitters such as serotonin and dopamine. Those who suffer from chronic pain and have few other treatment alternatives, as well as individuals recuperating from surgery who wish to speed up the healing process, may find this to be of particular use.

Does Not Require the Use of Drugs: PEMF therapy, on the other hand, does not include the use of any drugs or other kinds of medication in any way, therefore it is not to be confused with more traditional medical therapies. Instead, it makes use of the power that electromagnetic fields provide to directly activate cells in the body, which in turn helps the body recover itself.

This therapy is an alternative that is both secure and practical for individuals of any age because it does not involve the consumption of any medications or the performance of any intrusive procedures. PEMF therapy can give long-term comfort without the hazards that are connected with the use of prescription pharmaceuticals. This is true regardless of whether you are suffering from chronic pain, sleeplessness, or another illness.

Cons

More research is needed: Even though pulsed electromagnetic field treatment (PEMF) is successful in many instances, it is essential to keep in mind that further research is required to properly comprehend its effects and establish whether or not there are any feasible dangers associated with it. There have not been enough studies conducted over extended periods to demonstrate the safety and efficiency of PEMF therapy over the long term. This is because this kind of treatment has just lately acquired popularity.

Potential risks to people with certain conditions: In addition, several authorities in the field have voiced their worry about the potential for adverse effects on those who are affected by particular circumstances, such as those who are pregnant or who have a family history of cancer. To gain a better understanding of the potential effects that PEMF treatment may have on these populations and to determine whether any particular precautions should be taken, more study is required.

If you are thinking about undergoing PEMF therapy, it is imperative that you first consult with your primary care physician to have a comprehensive understanding of the therapy's possible negative effects as well as its potential advantages. You and your partner will be able to discuss the benefits and drawbacks of this treatment choice so that you can decide if it is appropriate for you.

Despite these drawbacks, a significant number of patients have discovered that pulsed electromagnetic field therapy (PEMF) can be a successful treatment choice for a wide variety of health disorders. PEMF should be considered as a potential alternative to more conventional forms of medical therapy for a variety of reasons, including postoperative recovery and the search for relief from persistent pain.

Side Effects of PEMF Therapy

Pulsed electromagnetic field therapy (PEMF therapy) is a well-liked alternative treatment that is reported to offer a wide variety of advantages, including the reduction of pain and inflammation as well as the improvement of circulation. Before beginning PEMF therapy, it is important to keep in mind that, just as with any other treatment, there is a possibility of experiencing adverse effects.

Headaches: Headaches are among the most often experienced adverse reactions to PEMF treatment. This is often because the magnetic fields employed in PEMF therapy can create changes in the activity level of the brain. If, after beginning PEMF therapy, you find that you are suffering from headaches, it is strongly suggested that you talk to your primary care physician about whether or not the treatment is appropriate for you.

Dizziness and nausea: Dizziness and nausea are two other symptoms that frequently accompany PEMF treatment. Changes in brain activity, including those that can induce headaches, are typically the root cause of this condition. If, after beginning PEMF therapy, you find that you are experiencing symptoms such as nausea or vertigo, it is strongly suggested that you talk to your primary care physician about whether or not you should continue with the treatment.

Fatigue: One of the potential negative effects of PEMF therapy is feeling tired all the time. In most cases, this is the result of the body's reaction to the magnetic fields that are utilized in the treatment. It is suggested that you speak with your physician if you are experiencing tiredness after beginning PEMF therapy to determine whether or not the therapy is appropriate for you.

Skin burns: PEMF treatment has been known to occasionally cause more serious adverse effects, including burns to the skin. In most cases, this is the result of coming into close touch with the magnetic field that is utilized in the treatment. If, after beginning PEMF therapy, you see burns on your skin, it is strongly suggested that you discuss the matter with your primary care physician to determine whether or not the treatment is appropriate for you.

If you start PEMF therapy and then notice any of these adverse effects, it is strongly suggested that you speak with your primary care physician about whether or not you should continue with the treatment.

Risks of PEMF Therapy

PEMF therapy is a relatively new treatment that is gaining in popularity for a wide range of ailments; nevertheless, before starting any treatment, it is essential to be informed of the potential side effects.

Even though pulsed electromagnetic field therapy is typically safe, there are a few potential hazards that patients should be aware of. These concerns include electrical shocks, seizures, cardiac rhythms, and interference with pacemakers. Let's take a more in-depth look at each of these potential risks.

Seizures: PEMF treatment has been linked to several significant adverse effects, including seizures, some of which can even be fatal. This disorder manifests itself when the brain's electrical impulses become imbalanced, causing the functioning of the brain to be disrupted and eventually leading to seizures. Convulsions, loss of consciousness, and a host of other symptoms, all of which call for prompt medical treatment, are possible manifestations of epileptic seizures.

In extremely rare instances, patients receiving PEMF therapy have reported experiencing seizures. These seizures often take place either during or soon after their treatment sessions. Because of this, it is essential for anybody who has a previous medical history of seizures to confer with their primary care physician before beginning PEMF therapy. This will assist in ensuring that any potential hazards may be recognized and mitigated to the greatest extent feasible.

Heart Arrhythmias: Arrhythmias of the heart should be kept in mind whenever one is weighing the advantages and disadvantages of PEMF therapy, as the possibility of these conditions should not be discounted. These irregular cardiac rhythms manifest themselves whenever the normal beating of the heart demonstrates an abnormality in either its rhythm or pace.

Atrial fibrillation and ventricular tachycardia are two typical examples of abnormal cardiac rhythms or arrhythmias. Problems with the electrical signals that govern the pulse, such as oxidative stress and damaged cell membranes, are often the root cause of irregular heart rhythms.

Even though some studies have demonstrated that PEMF therapy can be effective in reducing some of the symptoms that are associated with certain arrhythmias, further study is still required to fully understand how PEMF can impact these diseases.

In light of this information, anybody who is contemplating PEMF therapy should probably first speak with their primary care physician to evaluate whether or not they are at risk for cardiac arrhythmias and whether or not they would benefit from anti-arrhythmic drugs or other therapies. Before selecting whether or not pulsed electromagnetic field therapy (PEMF therapy) is the correct choice for you, it is essential to consider the possible advantages as well as the hazards.

Electrical Shocks: Because magnets may interact strongly with electrical circuits, this kind of treatment entails a minor danger of receiving an electric shock as a result of problems such as frayed cables or malfunctioning equipment. Physicians and other medical professionals must take appropriate safety measures before and during each PEMF therapy session to reduce the likelihood of adverse events and guarantee the well-being of patients undergoing the treatment. These processes can include testing the equipment before it is used, utilizing only the right materials during sessions, and verifying all wiring at various points throughout a patient's PEMF therapy.

Interference with Pacemakers: Another potential concern connected with PEMF therapy is that it might cause interference with pacemakers. There have been extremely rare instances of PEMF treatments causing problems with pacemakers, even though the risk is quite minimal. Before beginning PEMF therapy, you must discuss the matter with your physician if you are currently wearing a pacemaker.

Who Should Not Use PEMF Therapy?

Pregnant women or young children: It is recommended that pregnant women and children under the age of six stay away from PEMF therapy owing to safety concerns. Because there is currently a lack of clinical data about the impact that PEMF therapy can have on these groups, many healthcare providers prefer to err on the side of caution when it comes to treating their patients.

In addition to this, there is a worry that prenatal or pediatric treatment with PEMF might disrupt the natural development of the fetus or kid, resulting in long-term harm. Due to the presence of these dangers, it is strongly advised that expectant mothers and children under the age of 10 stay away from this particular form of therapy.

People with pacemakers or other implanted medical devices: It is crucial to be aware of the possible dangers connected with PEMF therapy if you have an implanted medical device such as a pacemaker or any other type of medical device. According to several studies, some varieties of electromagnetic fields have the potential to disrupt the typical operation of these devices, which might result in several undesirable side effects.

In addition, those who have any form of metal implant would wish to steer clear of PEMF therapy, as the devices used in this treatment might cause the implant to heat up. PEMF therapy, on the other hand, has the potential to offer several health advantages to patients suffering from a wide range of illnesses so long as it is administered correctly and under the supervision of a qualified medical expert. Therefore, if you are thinking of undergoing this kind of treatment, you should carefully examine the potential hazards versus the potential advantages of the treatment.

People with epilepsy: People who have epilepsy should exercise extreme caution if they are contemplating beginning a new treatment or therapy, as there is always the possibility that doing so might bring on a seizure. Because of this potential hazard, it is typically advised that epileptic patients refrain from receiving treatment using pulsed electromagnetic field (PEMF) devices.

Electrical currents are applied to the patient's body during PEMF therapy to speed up the healing process and lessen their level of discomfort. Those who have epilepsy are at risk of having seizure activity triggered by this substance due to its ability to both excite nerves and affect the functioning of the brain.

Anyone with a neurological condition: People who have other disorders that impact the nervous system, such as multiple sclerosis, should only utilize PEMF therapy under the advice of a specialist. This is because PEMF therapy affects the neurological activity that occurs throughout the body. Therefore, before beginning treatment with PEMF therapy, a person who has a neurological problem should carefully examine whether or not the therapy is appropriate for them.

People with cancer should consult a doctor first before starting this treatment: The application of pulsed electromagnetic field treatment (PEMF) to patients diagnosed with cancer is a contentious issue. Others contend that cancer patients should not utilize this therapy before first contacting a doctor, even though some experts feel that it can assist to relieve pain, stimulating wound healing, and boosting the effectiveness of drugs. This is because PEMF therapy might cause existing tumors to grow or spread more quickly, as well as conflict with other therapies now in use.

In addition to this, it has been demonstrated that it lowers the natural immunity of the body, which leaves patients more susceptible to infection and other severe health consequences. In the end, it is up to the individual patient to decide whether or not to participate in PEMF therapy; however, they are required to do so under the supervision of a trained medical practitioner.

Anyone who is thinking about undergoing PEMF therapy has to first consult with their primary care physician to determine whether or not it is appropriate for them.

A 5-Step Plan for Getting Started with PEMF

PEMF therapy is used by a lot of individuals because it helps ease pain, boosts circulation, and moves forward the healing process more quickly. If you're thinking about giving PEMF therapy a go, the following is a step-by-step guide to getting started with it.

Step 1: Determine If PEMF Therapy Is Right for You

It is crucial to do some study and figure out if pulsed electromagnetic field therapy (PEMF therapy) is the proper treatment for you before you begin using it. Have a discussion with your primary care provider to determine whether or not PEMF therapy is a viable treatment option for your unique medical problem. After you have made the decision that you wish to pursue PEMF therapy, the next step is to select the appropriate device.

Step 2: Choose the Right PEMF Device

When it comes to selecting a PEMF device, there are several considerations to take into account. You need to identify your budget first and foremost, and then you need to prioritize the many kinds of things that are vital to you.

Many individuals seek the advice of medical specialists, such as chiropractors and physical therapists, who are familiar with PEMF devices and may assist in pointing you in the direction of the solution that is most suited to meet your requirements.

You'll be able to start reaping the many rewards that come with undergoing PEMF therapy as soon as you've completed the necessary research and located a device that suits your requirements in terms of both its capabilities and its cost.

Step 3: Get Started With a PEMF Routine

The first thing you should do when you are ready to begin your PEMF program is to choose a posture in which you can feel most at ease. It is recommended that you lay down on your back and position the device so that it is either close to or directly over the portion of your body that you wish to concentrate on.

Alternately, you may begin by positioning the device over a bigger region, such as your entire spine or the area around your belly. This would be a good place to start. Relax and give the gadget some time to do its thing once you've established a comfortable posture and activated the device; at this point, all you need to do is sit back and let it do its thing. When undergoing PEMF therapy, it is not uncommon for patients to feel a tingling sensation throughout their bodies; however, this feeling should fade away after a few minutes of treatment.

As you move forward with your PEMF regimen, you should make an effort to avoid concentrating excessively on any sensations or feelings that may arise. Instead, you should make an effort to be in the here and now and be conscious of how you are feeling both physically and psychologically.

You will likely begin to see results in terms of improved energy levels and reduced pain or stress levels as time goes on and as you become more familiar with PEMF therapy and gain a better sense of what works best for both your body and mind. This will occur as you gain a better understanding of what works best for your body and mind.

Step 4: Listen to Your Body

Even while pulsed electromagnetic field treatment (PEMF) is usually believed to be safe, you must pay attention to your body and discontinue the use of the device if you experience any pain or discomfort. After utilizing a PEMF device, there is a possibility that some individuals can suffer from adverse effects like headaches or dizziness. These adverse effects are often modest and fleeting.

If you do encounter any adverse side effects, you should immediately cease using the device and speak with your primary care physician or another qualified medical professional.

Step 5: Re-Evaluate and Adjust As Necessary

When you've been engaging in PEMF therapy for a while, it's important to stop and assess how well it's working for you. Are you noticing any positive effects? Are there any potential drawbacks to this treatment? Make the necessary adjustments to your routine, and keep track of how the PEMF therapy is influencing your health.

Pulsed electromagnetic field therapy has the potential to be an efficient complementary and alternative treatment for a variety of different health issues. If you are thinking about giving PEMF therapy a go, the first thing you need to do is follow these five steps.

Picking the Perfect Pulsed Electromagnetic Field Therapy Device

Perhaps you've even given some thought to trying PEMF therapy, but you haven't been sure which device would be best for you. It might be difficult to know where to begin when there are so many various manufacturers and models available on the market. The following is a summary of everything that you need to think about when selecting a PEMF device for you to be able to make an educated choice that is suitable for you.

Price: When it comes to selecting a PEMF device, one of the first things you'll want to think about is how much money you're willing to spend on it. Because the price of PEMF therapy devices can range anywhere from a few hundred to several thousand dollars, it is essential to establish a budget before beginning your search for a device.

As soon as you have a crystal clear notion of how much money you are willing or able to spend, you will be able to reduce the number of possibilities available to you and concentrate on products that are priced within your budgetary constraints.

Features: When selecting a PEMF device, it is essential to take into account not only the device's fundamental capabilities but also its features and configurable options. Users can more readily target certain portions of their bodies or diseases when using certain devices that provide pulsed electromagnetic field treatment and are reasonably straightforward to operate.

However, other devices are more complete and come with extra capabilities that give you the ability to tailor your therapeutic experience to your specific needs. These more advanced features might include the ability to control the frequency and intensity of the pulses for more precise treatment, or they might include advanced tools like timers and memory channels that make it easier to save your preferred settings and switch between customized therapies at the touch of a button.

In the end, you should choose a PEMF device that provides the characteristics that are tailored to your requirements the best.

Ease of Use: When selecting a PEMF device, it is critical to think about not only how effective it is and what functions it has, but also how simple it is to operate. Because of how easy it is to set up and use some gadgets, they are perfect for people who have little to no prior experience working with technological equipment.

On the other hand, to correctly set up and operate other gadgets, you may need to expend more work or have more technical knowledge. If you are unsure of how comfortable you will be with new technology, it is in your best interest to select a tool that is not overly complicated and is easy to understand and operate.

Portability: If you want to use your PEMF device while traveling or when you are otherwise on the go, portability should be a primary concern for you. Some gadgets are small and compact enough to fit in carry-on luggage, whilst others are bulkier and require a specialized suitcase or duffel bag to carry them in. Think about how often you'll be using your gadget outside of the house, and pick one that's convenient to carry with you.

It is not necessary to have a tough time selecting the ideal Pulsed Electromagnetic Field Therapy gadget for your needs. If you only keep these things in mind, you'll have no trouble finding a piece of technology that works well for your needs.

Conclusion

The possible advantages of PEMF treatment are extensive and vary in nature. Some of the most important benefits include a reduction in pain and inflammation, as well as an improvement in blood circulation and the ability to repair damaged cells. PEMF therapy is a successful treatment for a broad variety of illnesses, including arthritis, migraine headaches, carpal tunnel syndrome, and chronic pain.

However, just like any other form of medical treatment, PEMF therapy is not without its share of potential side effects. To determine whether or not pulsed electromagnetic field therapy (PEMF therapy) is the appropriate kind of treatment for you, it is essential to first discuss your condition with a trained medical practitioner.

In general, pulsed electromagnetic field therapy (PEMF therapy) is a treatment that is both safe and effective, and it can give relief from a wide variety of illnesses. Discussing the potential benefits of PEMF therapy with your primary care physician or another qualified medical practitioner is a good first step if you are thinking about adopting this treatment option.

FAQ

1. What is PEMF therapy?

PEMF therapy is a type of therapy that uses pulsed electromagnetic fields to stimulate healing. The therapy is based on the principle that all cells in the body have an electromagnetic field, and that this field can be used to promote healing.

2. How does PEMF therapy work?

PEMF therapy works by delivering pulses of electromagnetic energy to the body. These pulses stimulate the cells and help to promote healing.

3. What are the benefits of PEMF therapy?

PEMF therapy is effective for a variety of conditions, including pain relief, wound healing, and tissue regeneration. Additionally, PEMF therapy has been shown to improve circulation and increase cell oxygenation.

4. Are there any side effects associated with PEMF therapy?

PEMF therapy is generally considered to be safe, with few side effects reported. The most common side effect is mild skin irritation, which typically resolves within a few days.

5. How long does PEMF therapy take?

PEMF therapy sessions typically last between 30 and 60 minutes. However, some people may require multiple sessions per day or week to achieve desired results.

6. How often does PEMF therapy need to be done?

PEMF therapy is typically done daily, although some people may only require it once or twice per week. Maintenance sessions may also be required once results have been achieved to prevent relapse.

7. Is PEMF therapy covered by insurance?

PEMF therapy is not typically covered by insurance, as it is considered to be an experimental treatment. However, some insurance companies may cover the cost of PEMF devices if they are medically necessary for the treatment of a specific condition.

8. How much does PEMF therapy cost?

The cost of PEMF therapy can vary depending on the type of device used and the number of sessions required. Typically, a single session will cost between $50 and $100, although discounts may be available if multiple sessions are purchased in advance.

References and Helpful Links

5 best PEMF therapy devices & how to choose one. (2022, August 18). Healthline. https://www.healthline.com/health/pemf-therapy-device.

MD, C. H. R. (2015). Use of pulsed electromagnetic fields in reducing arm and shoulder complaints in breast cancer patients after lymph node dissection (Clinical Trial Registration No. NCT01255631). clinicaltrials.gov. https://clinicaltrials.gov/ct2/show/NCT01255631.

PEMF therapy—Frequently asked questions. (2019, October 29). I-Tech Medical Division. https://itechmedicaldivision.com/en/pemf-therapy-frequently-asked-questions/.

Pulsed electromagnetic field therapy: Innovative treatment for diabetic neuropathy. (n.d.). Retrieved October 28, 2022, from https://www.practicalpainmanagement.com/treatments/interventional/stimulators/pulsed-electromagnetic-field-therapy-innovative-treatment.

The complete guide to PEMF therapy. (n.d.). Chiropractic Economics. Retrieved October 28, 2022, from https://www.chiroeco.com/complete-guide-pemf-therapy/.

What are the benefits of pulse PEMF therapy? (n.d.). Retrieved October 28, 2022, from https://ioaregenerative.com/blog/what-are-the-benefits-of-pulse-pemf-therapy.

Printed in the USA
CPSIA information can be obtained
at www.ICGtesting.com
LVHW011935050124
768156LV00001B/283